BUZZ TO BUZZKILL

How Alcohol and Dopamine Hack Your Brain

By Annie Grace
Illustrated by Mary Purdie

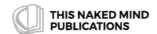

THIS NAKED MIND PUBLICATIONS

PRAISE FOR *BUZZ TO BUZZKILL*

"It's a great book. It tells me a lot about alcohol. And will really help me in the future."
—Trace, 11

"The brain is so interesting, and definitely not made for alcohol!"
—Lana, 16

"So interesting; why does anyone drink? And why don't they teach us this in school?"
—Turner, 13

"This book is great, unlike alcohol."
—Jayla, 13

Published and distributed by This Naked Mind
Publications in Boulder, Colorado
www.thisnakedmindpublications.com

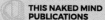

THIS NAKED MIND
PUBLICATIONS

Library of Congress Control Number: 2022908957
ISBN 978-0-9967150-5-8 (paperback)
ISBN 978-0-9967150-6-5 (EPUB)

Editor: Allison Serrell
Cover and interior illustrator: Mary Purdie
Cover and interior design: Tim Palin Creative
Author photo: Megan Hoffer

Produced by Wonderwell
www.wonderwell.press

WONDERWELL

Printed and bound in the US

To Turner, Trace, Daelyn, Lana, Jayla & Ki— let's make a better world together.

Thank you to my incredible illustrator, Mary Purdie.

AUTHOR'S DISCLAIMER

The author is not engaged in rendering professional advice or services to the individual readers. This work is a synthesis of scientific information, gathered from many sources and articulated in story form, for the purpose of understanding and consumption by people of all ages, with a special focus on younger humans. The ideas, procedures, and suggestions contained in this book are not intended as a substitute for consulting with your physician. All matters regarding your health require medical supervision. The author shall not be liable or responsible for any loss or damage allegedly arising from any information or suggestion in this book. If you feel you need more help with drinking, please visit ThisNakedMind.com or join us for a Free 30-Day Alcohol-Free Challenge at AlcoholExperiment.com.

CONTENTS

AUTHOR'S NOTE

I created This Naked Mind based on my own journey. In my 30s, I realized I was drinking too much, but nothing really *bad* had ever happened, and I didn't want to have to call myself an "alcoholic" to change my drinking habits. I started to research alcohol to find out why I was drinking more than I ever intended, and what I found really surprised me. I learned that many people don't fully understand how alcohol affects them, even though they drink it regularly.

If you want to dive deep into the research, it is available for free at AlcoholExperiment.com, but for now I'll share the most important things I learned:

1. Self-compassion (being nice to yourself instead of blaming and shaming) is actually one of the most productive ways to change an unhealthy habit. *This goes for anything, not just drinking.*

2. The term *alcoholic* seems to do more harm than good (it causes more shame and blame) and is not even scientifically or medically accurate.

3.   Instead of asking ourselves "What's wrong with me?" or "Do I have a problem?" I found a far more productive question to ask was "Would my life be better without alcohol?" Our brains kinda behave like Google—when we ask a question, the answer comes automatically. The same happens when we ask negative questions like "What's wrong with me?" This taught me to be thoughtful with the questions I asked myself, not only about alcohol but about everything.

This book was written with my kids in mind but the message is relevant for everyone. Young, old, in between. Anyone who is or will be exposed to alcohol. It explains the four main things that I wish I had known before I picked up a drink. While I am grateful for my journey, even the hard and messy parts, I do believe it would have been less painful if I had known these things *before* I started drinking.

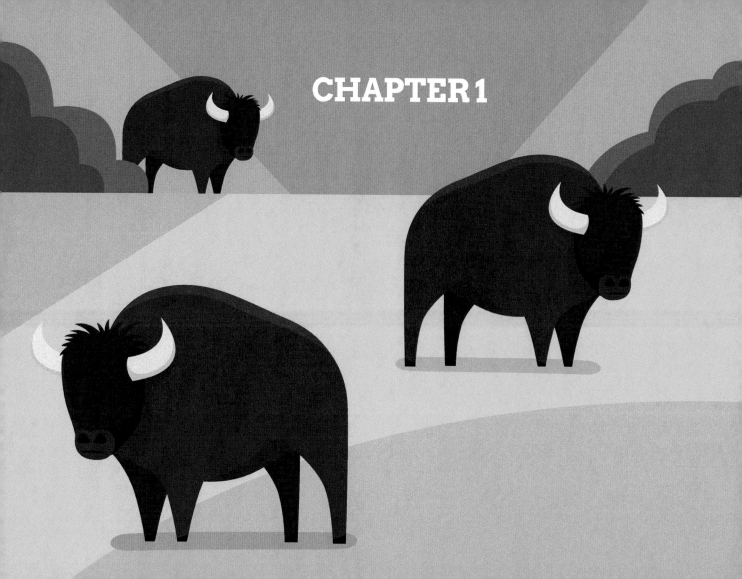

CHAPTER 1

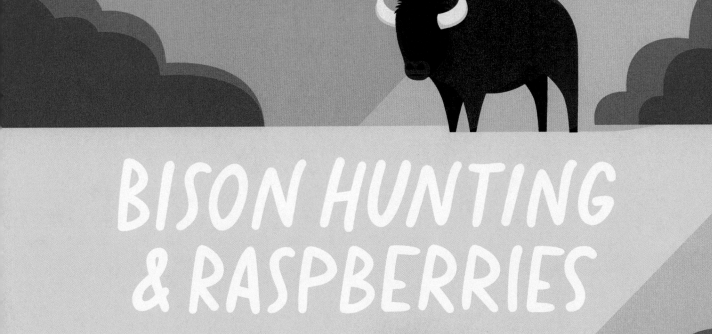

BISON HUNTING
& RASPBERRIES

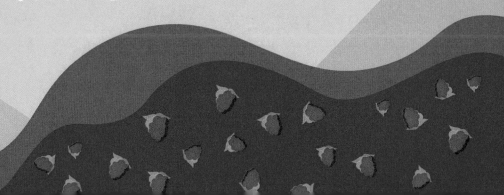

Imagine living back in the Stone Age and trying to survive without the internet or a grocery store. Sound terrible to you, too?

Great news! Your brain is a survival machine! One of the ways the brain helps us survive is by producing dopamine.

Dopamine is a neurotransmitter.
Neuro = Brain
Transmitter = Mover of information

Dopamine makes us do stuff.

So, you're a hunter-gatherer in the Stone Age, looking for food. You find a wild raspberry bush and gather the berries.

Your brain lights up and, you guessed it, releases *dopamine*.

Dopamine says, "Yes! Raspberries are good! They will help us survive. Let's *remember* raspberries."

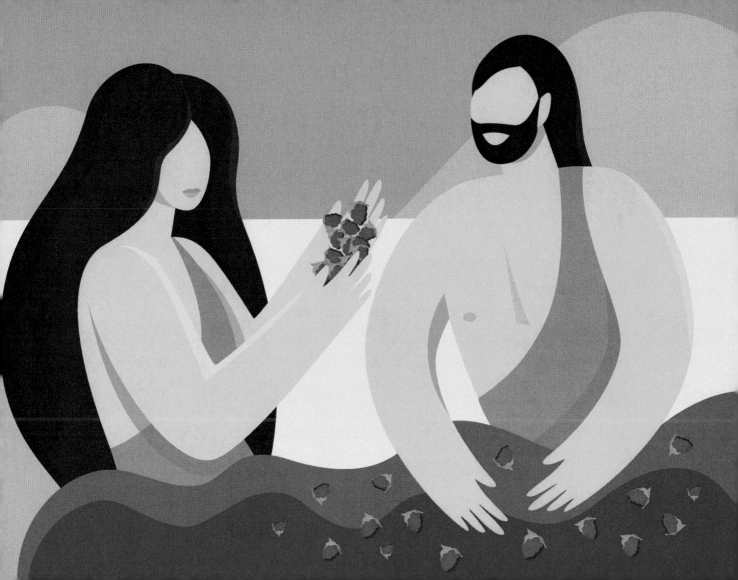

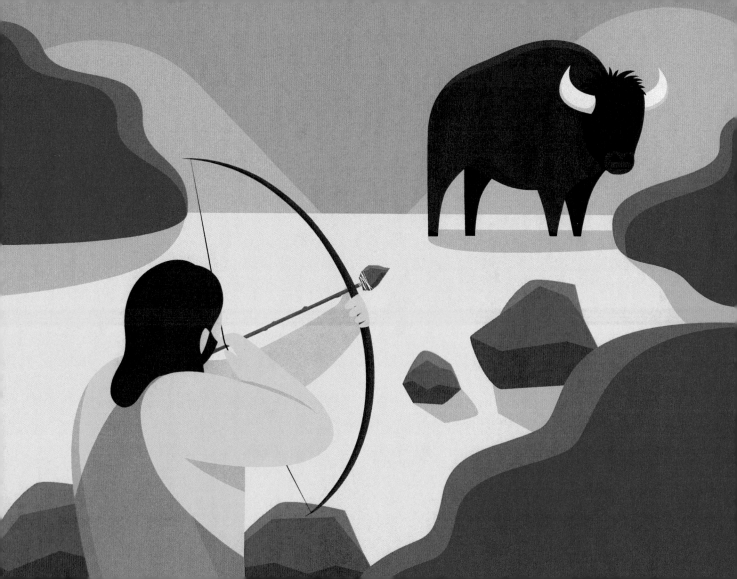

The brain produces dopamine when it thinks it's found something that will help you survive. Like raspberries.

Or, take bison hunting. In the Stone Age, our brains released dopamine to trigger a nice feeling when we hit our target—bison for dinner, anyone?

Finding and eating wild raspberries *feels good*.
Hitting a target while hunting *feels good*.
And so, we want to do these things again. And again… and again…

Your brain knows it's easier to do something when you *want to do it*.
So, dopamine creates that desire—*wanting*.

Most of us don't hunt bison anymore, but we experience that same good feeling—the rush of hitting a target—when we play video games.

It *feels good* to hit targets in a game.

That's dopamine.

But instead of just occasionally hitting a target, like when hunting, we can hit targets hundreds of times per minute playing video games.

Dopamine. Dopamine. Dopamine. Dopamine.
Extra dopamine.

Artificially high levels of dopamine (*artificial* just means not found in nature).

So, what's the problem? Here's where it gets interesting.

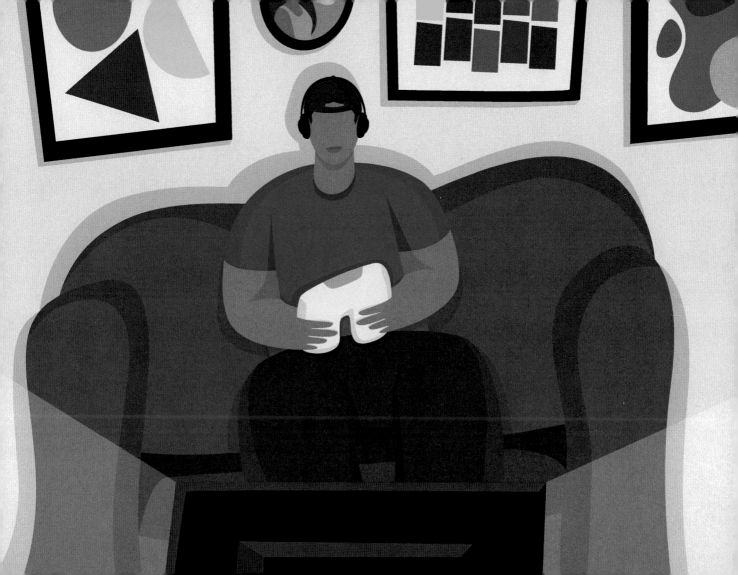

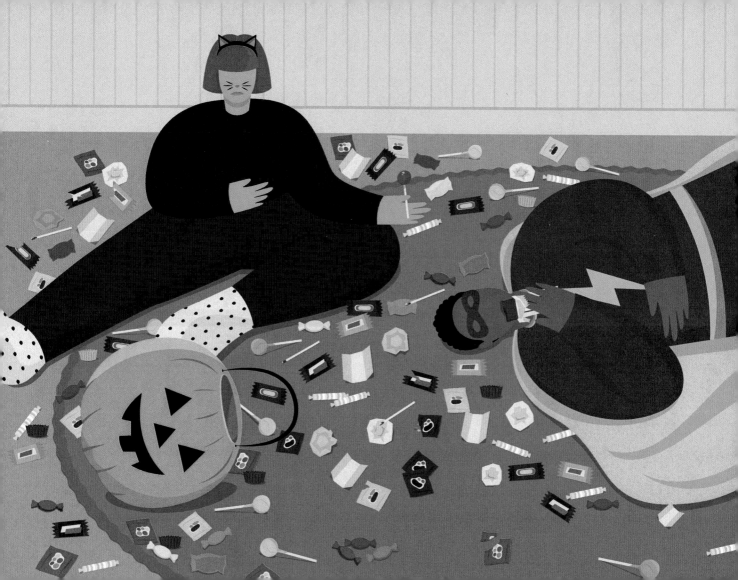

Dopamine creates desire—*wanting*.

But not necessarily enjoyment—*liking*.

So, you end up really *wanting* to do something you might not even *like*.

Say what?

Maybe you've experienced this.

Think of a time when you were younger, and you ate a ton of Halloween candy—so much candy that it stopped tasting good and you felt sick.

But some part of you still *wanted* to eat the candy—even when it wasn't fun anymore.

You wanted it, but you no longer liked it.

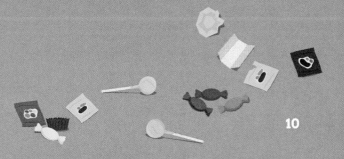

Why did you eat more than you enjoyed? Dopamine!

Dopamine makes you believe you still want it even after you no longer like it.

While raspberries create a normal "yes, this is good, let's do it again" response from your brain, candy *changes your dopamine system. It triggers so much dopamine that it hacks your brain.*

Or maybe, more recently, you were playing a video game or scrolling TikTok all weekend or over the summer. By the end of the day, you probably got sick of it, but you kept staring at the screen anyway.

Why did you keep playing the game or watching videos, even when you were tired of it?

You guessed it! Dopamine hacked your brain.

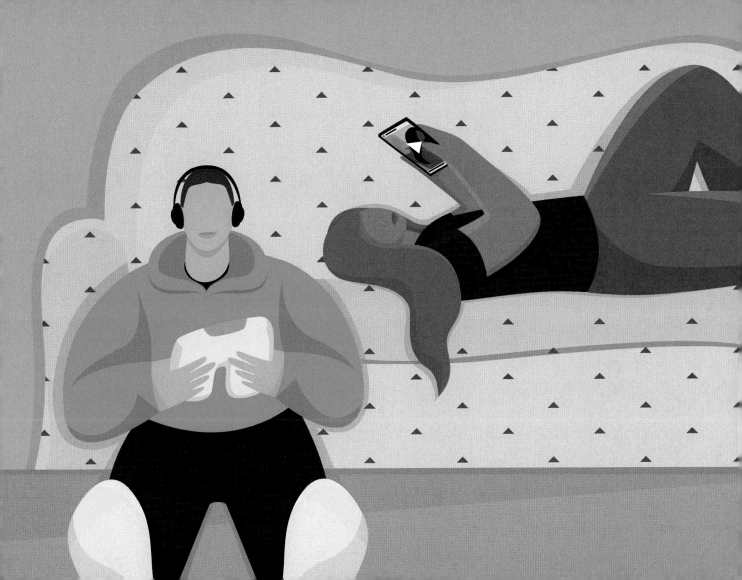

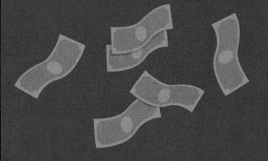

In fact, all addictive substances do this.

From heroin to alcohol, video games to processed sugar.

They all hack your brain by creating artificially high levels of dopamine.

And guess what else addictive substances have in common?

Profit. Dollars.

Someone somewhere is making *a lot of money* hacking your brain—selling you stuff that will make you want more and more, even after you stop liking it.

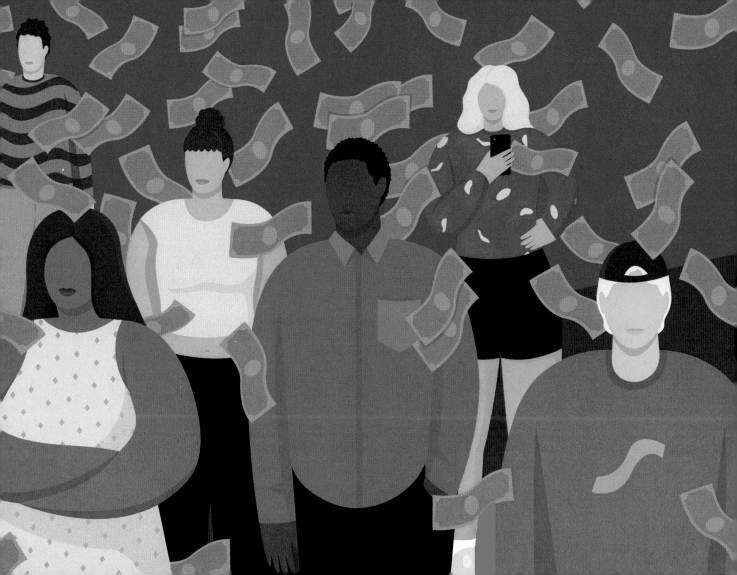

Alcohol makes our dopamine levels go especially wild, so it doesn't even matter if it tastes bad (my first taste was *gross*; I spit it out) or if the feeling isn't all that fun (I just felt dizzy).

Our brains can learn...

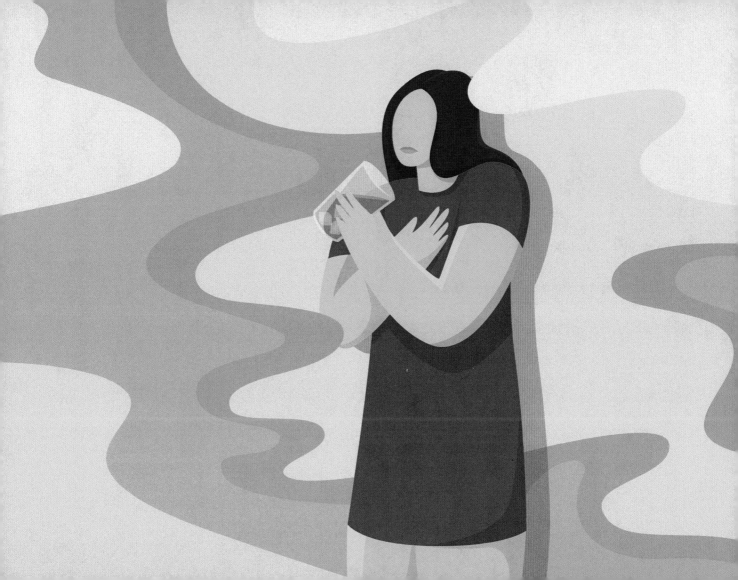

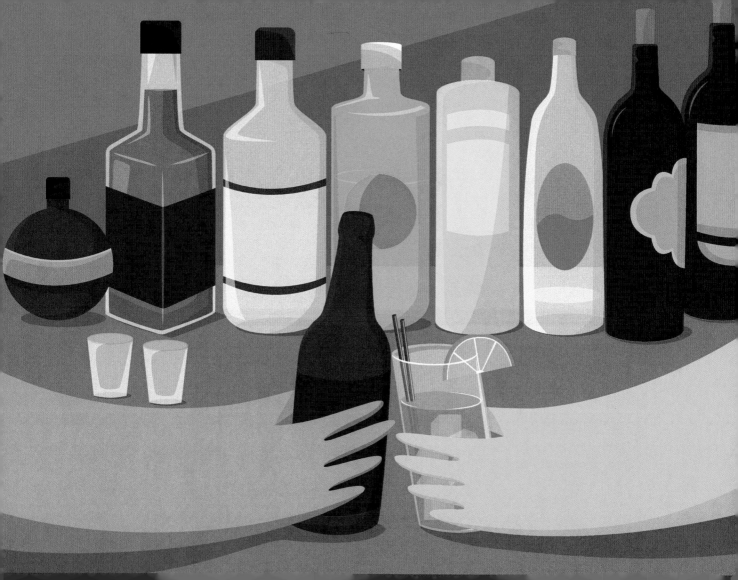

And the brain decides alcohol is important.

The brain—our body's survival machine—gets the message that we *need* to drink more *in order to survive*.

Eventually, alcohol tricks your brain into believing you ***cannot survive without it***.

So, when you drink, even if you don't really like it, the alcohol is slowly hacking your brain, telling you to do it again.

And again.

And again.

Alcohol is addictive.

Not just to some humans—to all humans. (At least any human with a brain.)

And *a lot* of money is spent advertising alcohol, especially toward younger people.

Because companies know—the sooner they get you to drink, the sooner your brain will believe it needs alcohol.

And the more money they will make.

That's something I wish I had known before my first drink.[12]

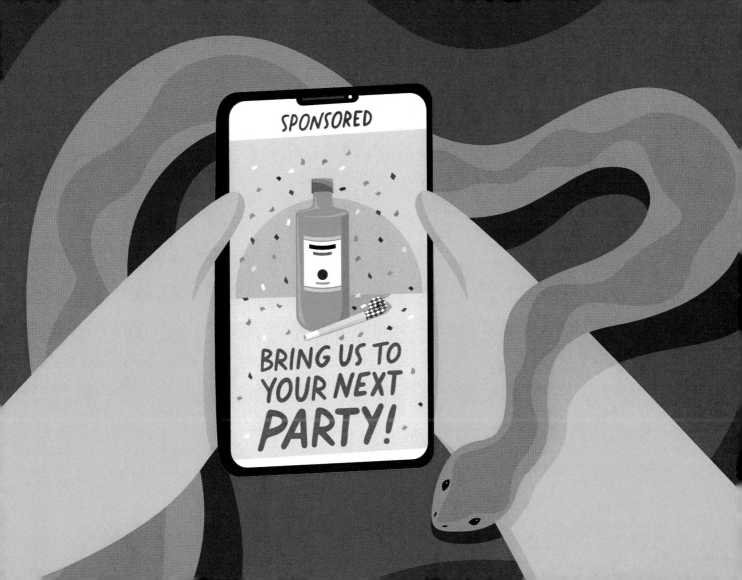

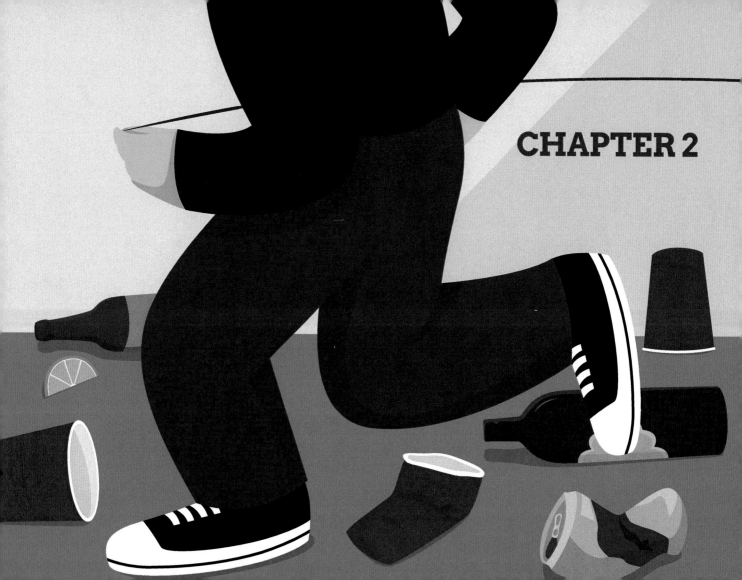

CHAPTER 2

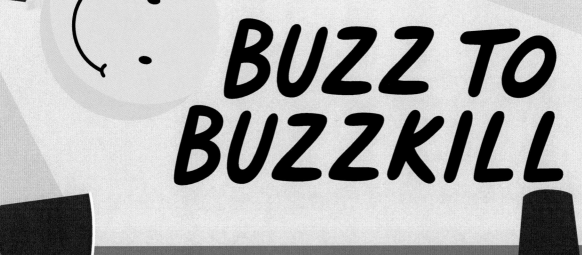
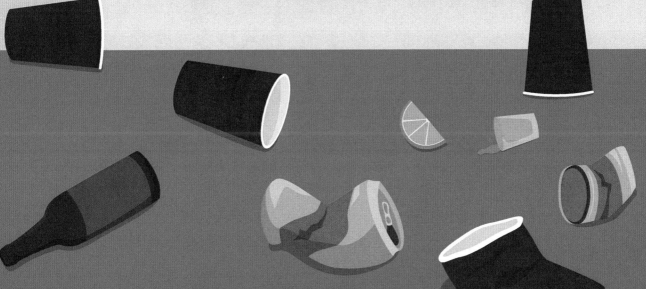

BUZZ TO
BUZZKILL

But wait, don't people drink because it *feels good, gives them a buzz*?

Well, sorta.

In fact, that's part of what gets us stuck—these temporary feelings.

Alcohol actually *overstimulates* the pleasure circuits in the brain, or the "feel good" parts of the brain. Kinda sounds like the whole point, right? People drink because it feels good?

But there's a problem. A **big** one.

Let me explain.

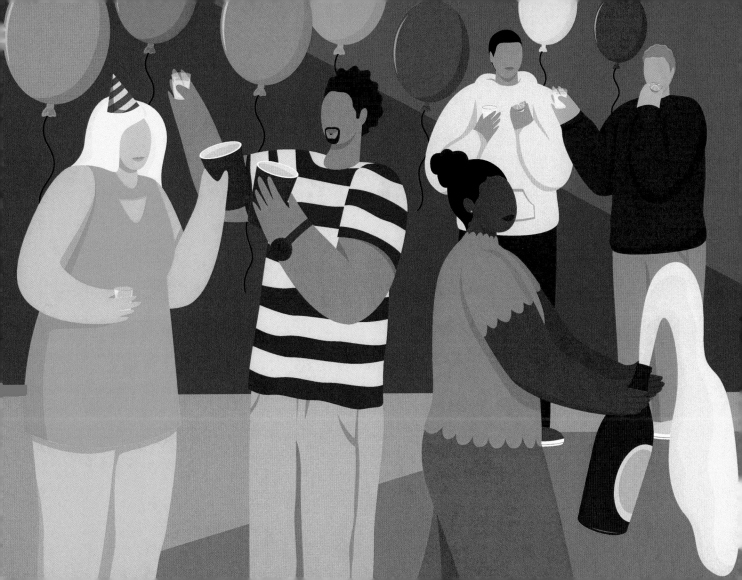

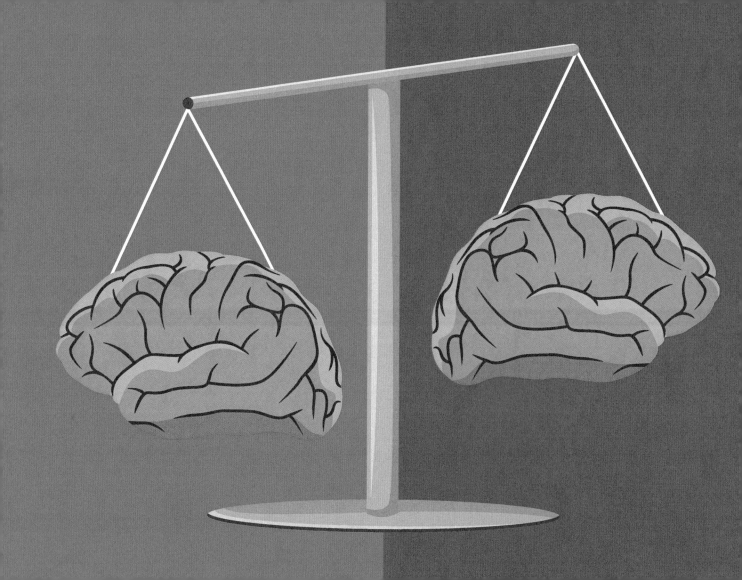

First, we need to learn about homeostasis.

Homeostasis means "finding stability" or "staying in balance."

Homeostasis is one of the ways your brain keeps you alive, safe, and feeling good.

Your brain is arguably the most complex organ in the known universe.

And like any amazing technology, it needs proper conditions to function well.

Kinda like how phones start glitching if they get too hot, the brain needs stability. Balance. *Homeostasis*.

Homeostasis is why you sweat. When your body gets too hot, it sweats to cool you down. Your body goes out of balance (too hot), and the sweat helps bring your body back into balance (the sweat evaporates, and your body cools down).

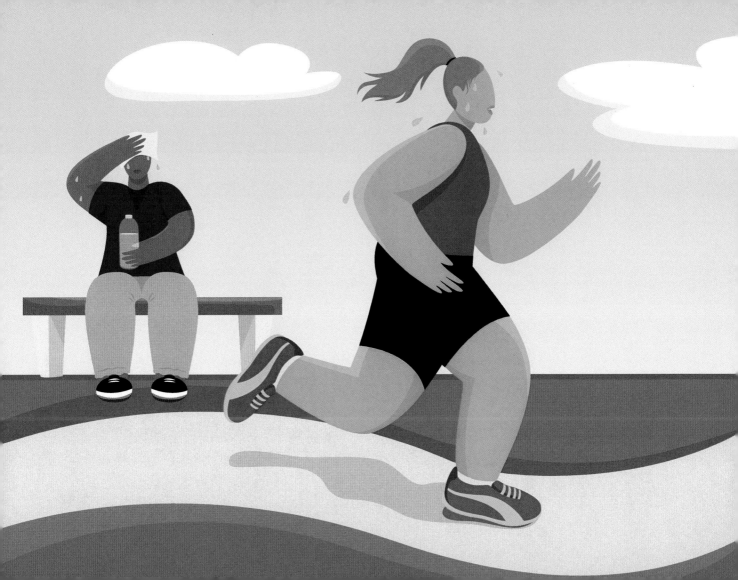

When the brain's pleasure center is overstimulated—*like when you drink alcohol*—the brain must do something to regain balance.

But how? Well, sometimes the brain creates chemicals.

Not the chemicals you use in a science lab, but natural chemicals that change things inside your brain and body.

Dynorphin is one of these chemicals (technically it's called a *peptide*).

Dynorphin can change how you feel.

And—spoiler alert—dynorphin makes you feel bad.[3]

Weird, right?

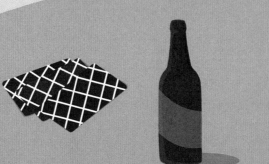

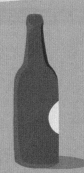

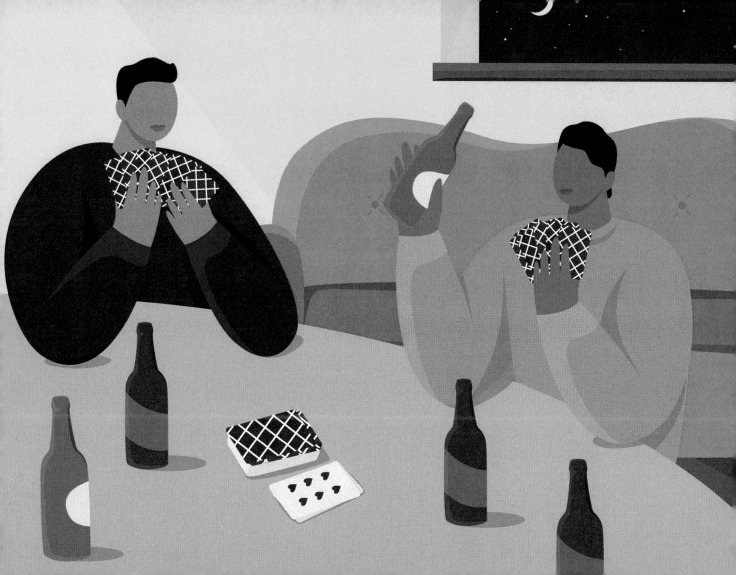

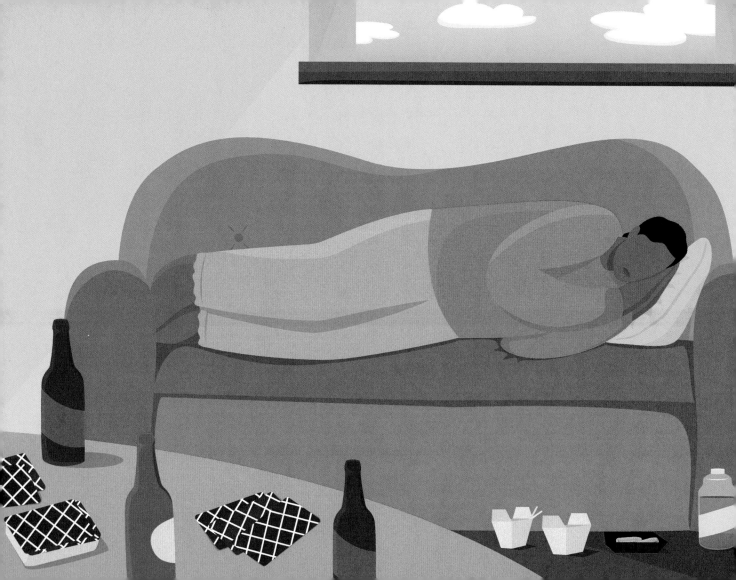

If alcohol makes your brain *feel good*, why would your brain respond by making you *feel bad*?

Homeostasis—to bring things back into balance.

This *only* happens when the brain determines it's experiencing something disruptive—*unsafe*.

And don't worry—this doesn't happen when you feel pleasure naturally, when you're just having fun.

So, alcohol makes you feel good (at least for a little while), but then dynorphin makes that vibe go away. No big deal, right?

Wrong. Here's why.

Alcohol is toxic to the human body. The alcohol we drink is actually a type of alcohol called ethanol.

You may have heard of ethanol—at the gas station.

Yep, ethanol is found in gasoline.

The same stuff you put in your car. Yes, the stuff with all the warnings like "don't inhale" and "toxic if ingested."

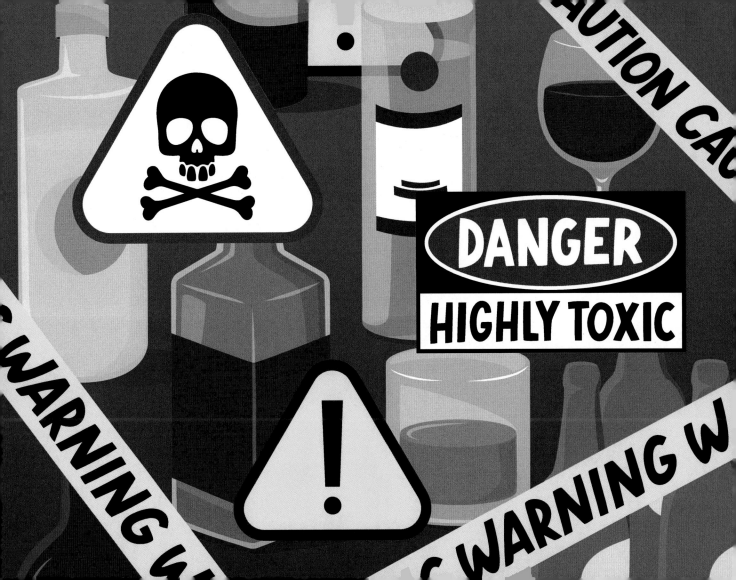

Why do adults drink something if it's so toxic? Partially because of the temporary pleasure. Partially because they don't realize how toxic it is. Partially because everyone's doing it. And partially because more than two billion dollars are spent every year, in the US alone, on advertising to convince us that we need alcohol.[4] That alcohol is fun and vital to adulthood. Vital to a good life.

If you give mice alcohol, they won't drink it. They might smell it or taste it, but their little mice brains tell them, "Poison! Stay away!" And since big companies aren't advertising it to them, and society isn't pressuring them, they trust their instincts.

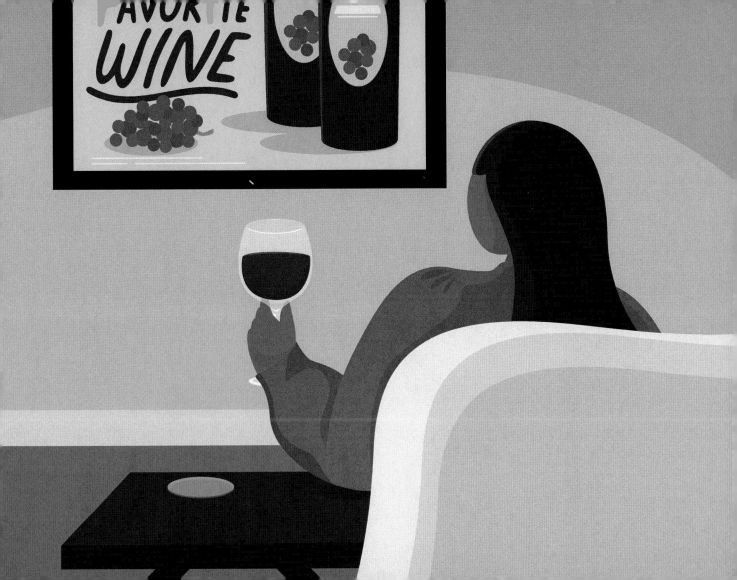

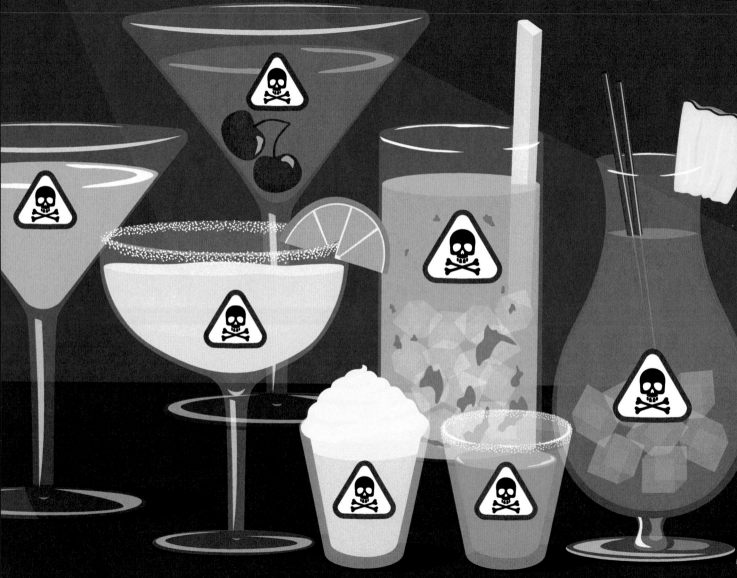

We humans ignore this instinct and do all sorts of things to make alcohol taste good enough to drink.

We have distilling processes and sugary mixers.

We water it down and sweeten it.

We do all this so we can drink it without immediately throwing up (which would happen if you drank pure alcohol).

Actually, just a little pure alcohol would kill you. Even watered-down alcohol kills more than twice as many people as drugs do every year.[56]

Even though we've figured out a way to make ethanol drinkable, it's still toxic.

Our taste buds can be fooled, but our bodies know the truth.

As soon as alcohol enters the system, the body goes on red alert and tries to get rid of the poison.

In fact, this job—kicking out the alcohol—is so important, the body will actually stop doing other things like digesting food or maintaining your blood sugar levels (a guaranteed recipe to make you *hangry*), in order to focus all its efforts on the alcohol.

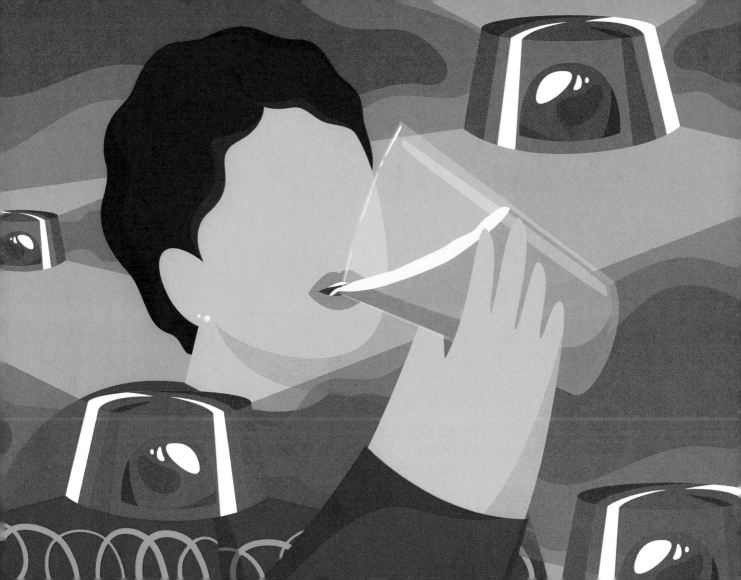

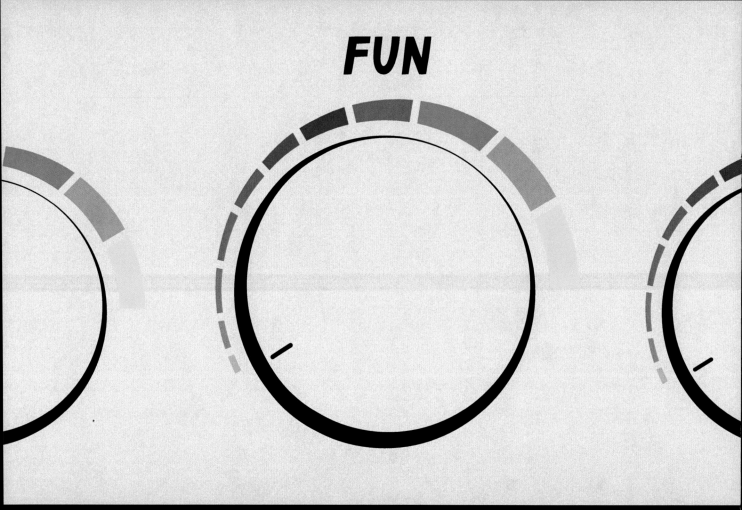

The body gets rid of the alcohol—and finally chills out.

But the other chemical, the one your brain produced to offset the alcohol? Dynorphin? It's not toxic. In fact, it was produced by your body in the first place, so there's no reason for the body to get rid of it.

Remember, dynorphin's job is to *turn down* pleasure—to make things less fun. But it doesn't just turn down pleasure from alcohol.

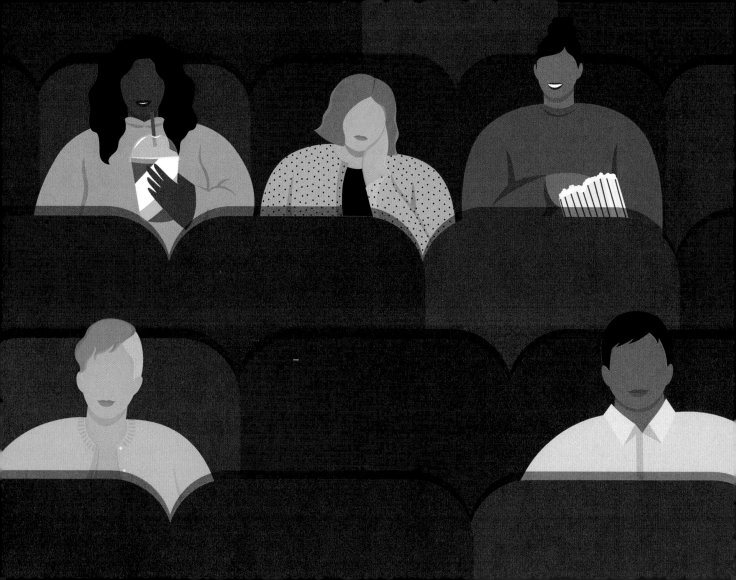

Dynorphin turns down all sorts of pleasure and makes it harder to enjoy everyday things:

- Hanging out with friends

- Reading a good book

- Watching a movie or a sports game

Interesting fact:
Drinking also causes the body to release stress hormones (like cortisol). If you're anxious already, drinking alcohol is like turning your anxiety up, literally increasing the anxiety and sadness you already feel. But a lot of people don't realize this because they don't feel their anxiety spike as soon as they take a drink—that feeling comes in the hours and days afterward.

And you start to wonder why life just kinda sucks, or why you feel anxious all the time.

You may have heard people say that they can't really have fun without a drink.

Sadly, that can become true.

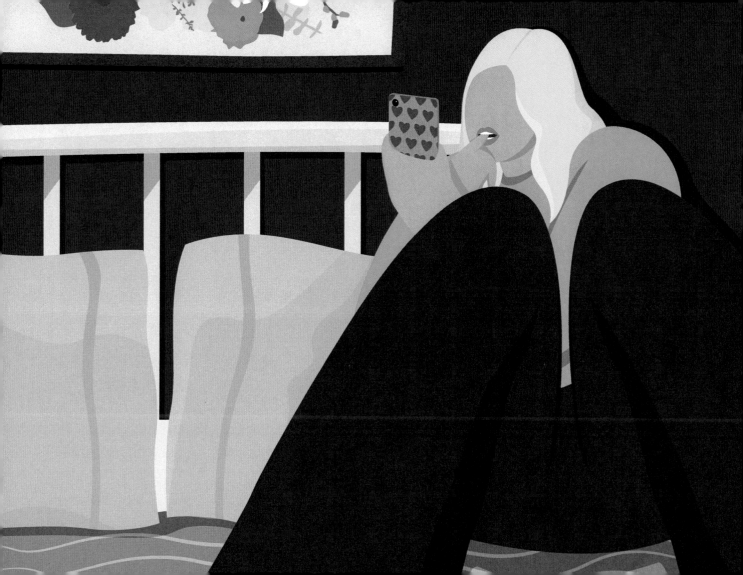

But it's not that you can't have fun without a drink—in fact, the science shows that things are often *more fun* without drinking.[7]

It's that the dynorphin stays in your body a lot longer than alcohol does, making it harder to experience fun naturally.

And over time, even the fun you get from drinking lessens.

And lessens.

And lessens.

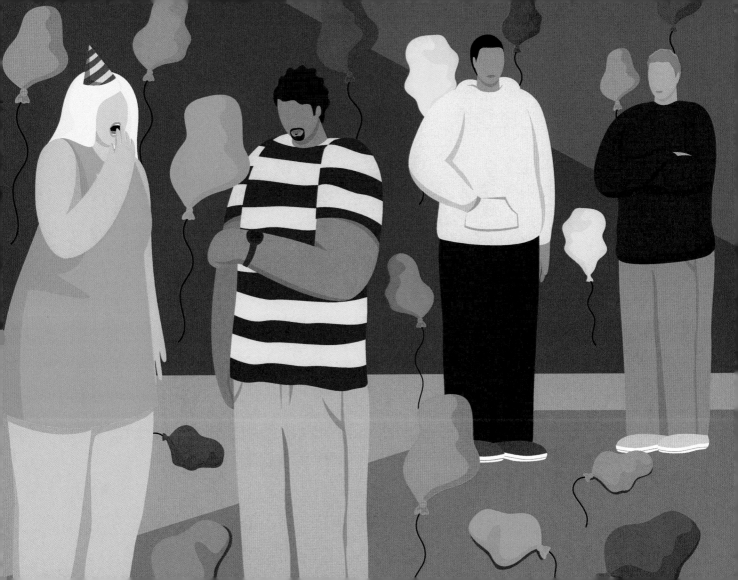

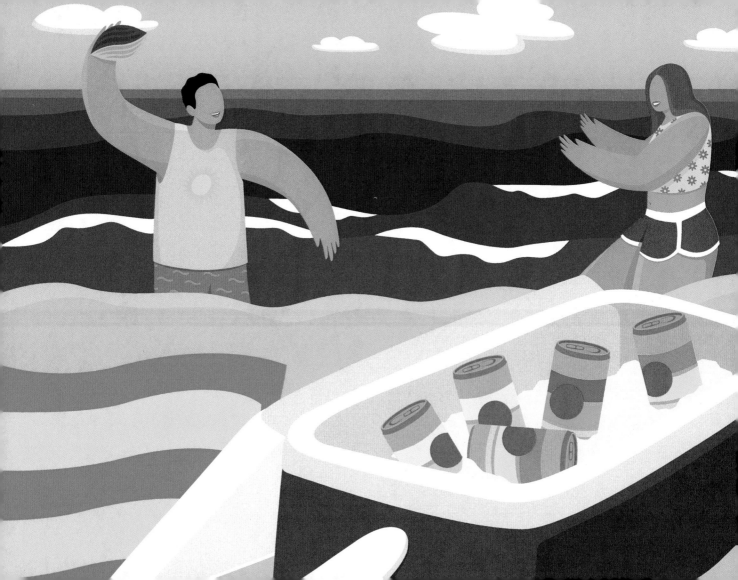

At the same time, the fun you get from all the other things in your life—things that aren't about drinking—also lessens and lessens and lessens.

Think of a great time you had hanging out with your friends.

With no alcohol, hanging out with your friends might be an 8 out of 10 on the fun scale.

You have a drink, and for a short period of time (more on that later), it becomes a 9 out of 10. That's the artificial stimulation of the pleasure center of your brain.

Then dynorphin kicks in, turning down your fun.

The next day, you're with your friends, not drinking—the fun is a 7 out of 10.

So, you drink. But the drink only brings you to an 8 out of 10 (which, by the way, is where you started).

The day after that, because of dynorphin still being in your body, the fun is a 6 out of 10. So, you drink.

And the drink brings you to a 7 out of 10.

Do you see where this is going?

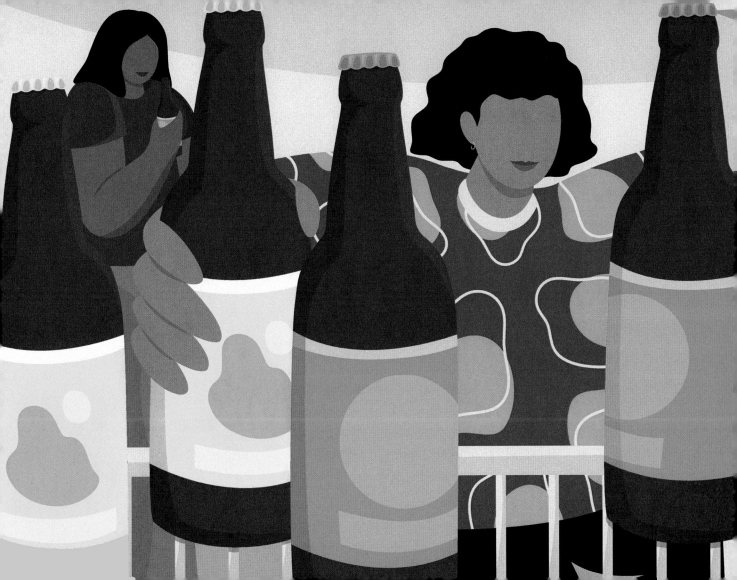

Eventually, hanging out with your friends without drinking isn't fun.

And

Eventually, hanging out with your friends—even when drinking—is no longer fun.

This takes some time but the pattern is the same.

It's called the law of diminishing returns, which basically means that, yes, alcohol will pick you up—a bit. But then it kicks you down further than you were before you drank. And even drinking again won't bring you back up to *your normal level of fun*!

Or, said another way: Alcohol will kick-start your anxiety and steal your joy.

Alcohol is the thief of joy.

And that's something I wish I had known before I had my first drink.[8][9]

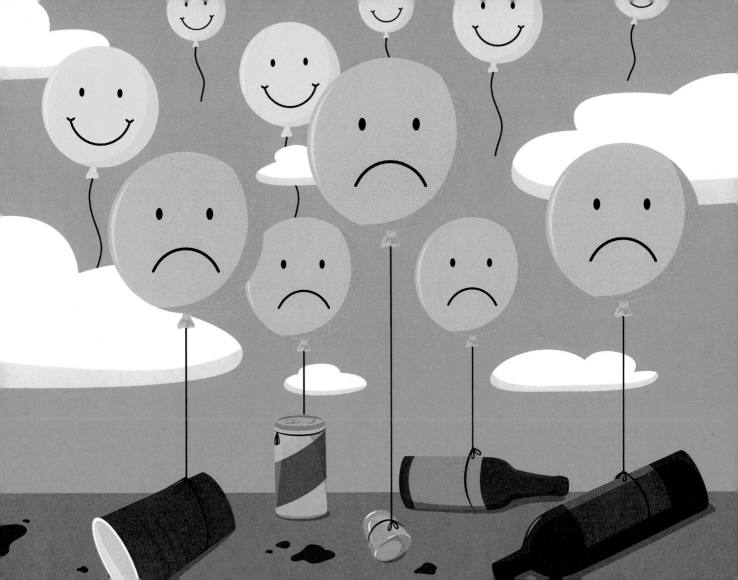

CHAPTER 3

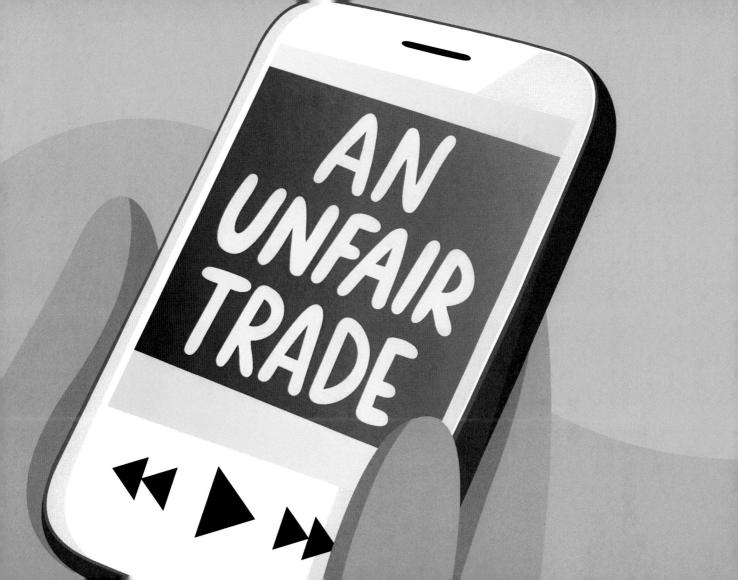

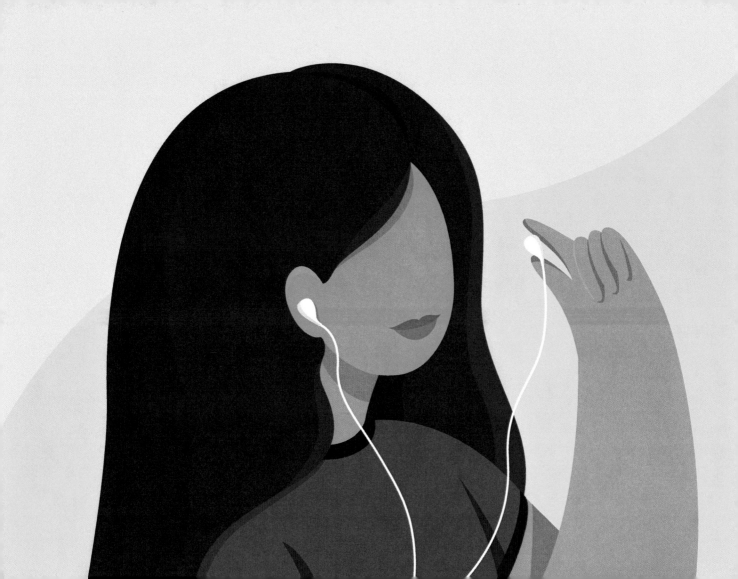

Would you trade 20 minutes of listening to your favorite music for 2–3 hours of listening to a song you hate on repeat?

Stupid question, right?

But that's what drinkers do all the time—just in a different way.

Let me explain.

Alcohol is both a stimulant and a depressant.

Stimulant = Gives your body more energy
Depressant = Takes away your energy

When you first drink alcohol, it makes its way into your blood—and it makes your blood alcohol content rise.

Like we already talked about, there are some good feelings associated with your blood alcohol levels rising. (That's part of the reason people drink in the first place.)

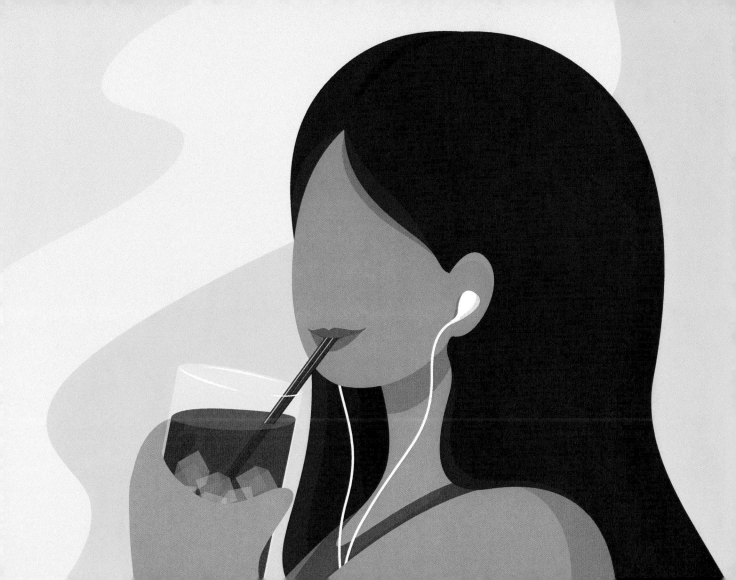

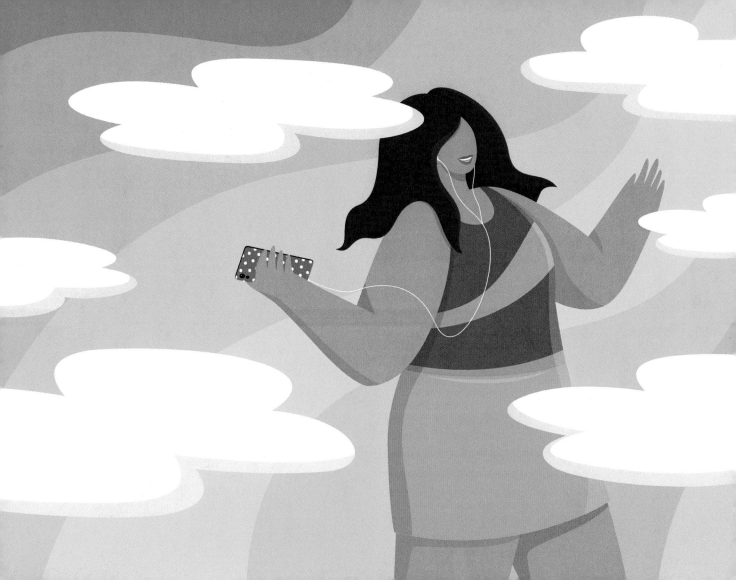

At this stage of drinking, alcohol acts as a stimulant.

You feel a bit more energy.

Kinda dizzy.
Light-headed.
The "buzz."

But since alcohol is toxic, the body says, "Intruder! Alert!" and rushes to get rid of the alcohol as quickly as possible.

In a very short amount of time—about 20 minutes—your blood alcohol content starts *decreasing*.

This is where alcohol becomes the worst.

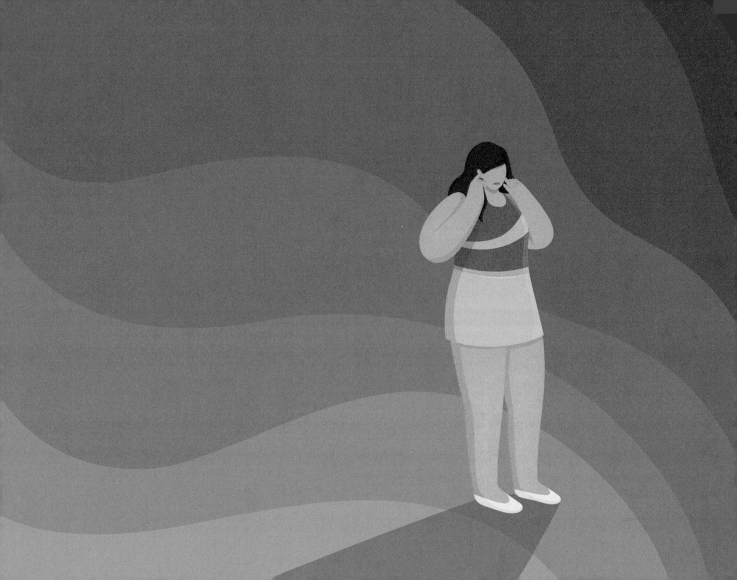

If you notice that *depressant* sounds a lot like *depressed*, you're right—it's the same type of feeling.

When your blood alcohol is falling, you experience all sorts of unpleasant feelings.

You'll feel uneasy.
Tired.
Anxious.
Uncomfortable.
Upset.
Sad.
Stressed.

And those feelings last a loooong time.

After one drink, you might have 18–20 minutes of nice feelings—immediately followed by 2–3 hours of not-so-nice feelings.

But we don't really notice it.

We don't connect the negative feeling with alcohol—it made us feel good, so we assume we're just stressed.

Also, as soon as we start to feel bad, we reach for another drink, trying to keep the good feelings going.

In my experience, I never quite got the same feeling with drink 2 or 3 as I did with that first drink.

Even though I tried, a lot.

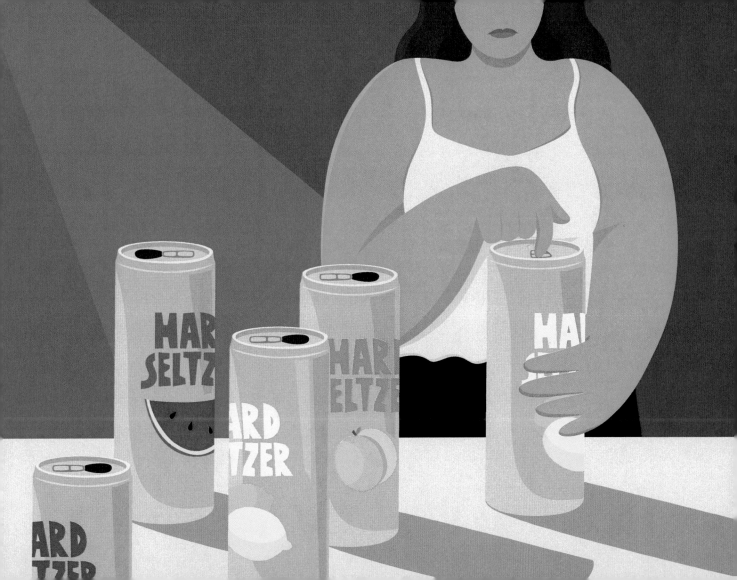

So, 20 minutes of fun for 2–3 hours of depressed feelings?

Now that's an unfair trade.

And something I wish I had known before my first drink.

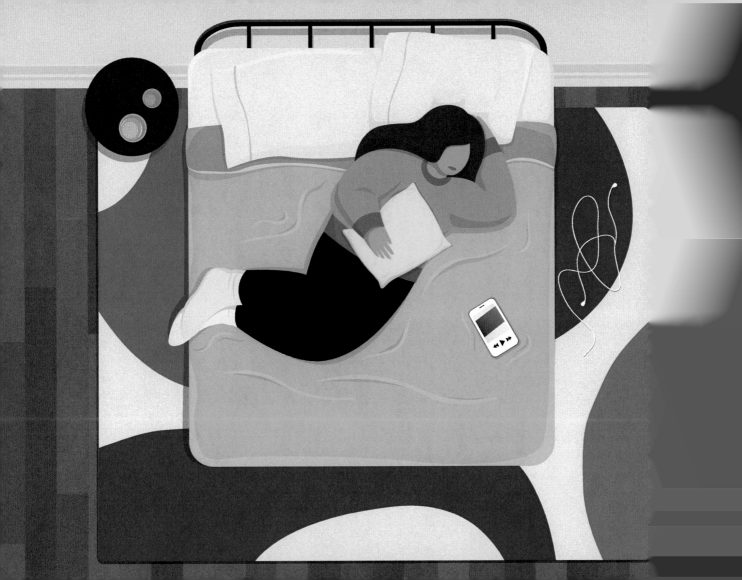

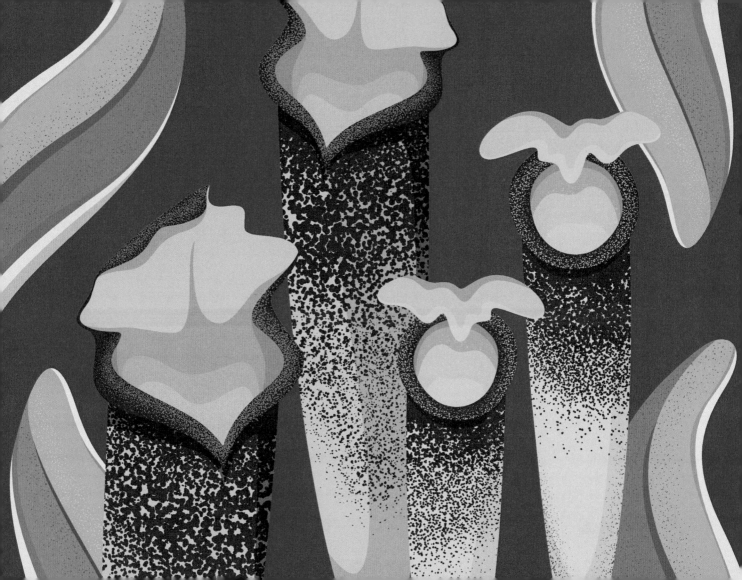

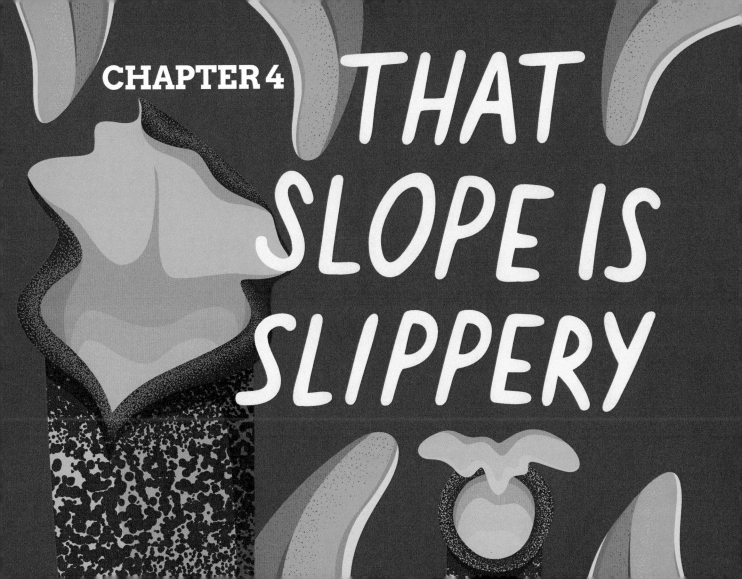

CHAPTER 4

THAT SLOPE IS SLIPPERY

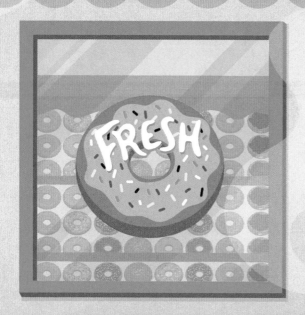
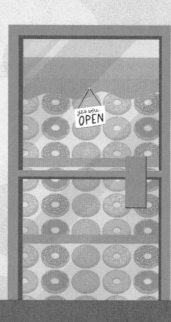
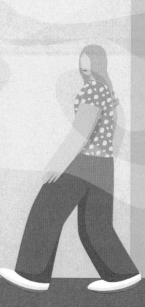

The best way I've ever heard the slide into alcohol explained is by the late author Allen Carr (RIP).

Imagine you're walking by your favorite doughnut shop, and you smell the delicious, fresh doughnuts and sugary sweet glaze. Your mouth waters, and you suddenly want a doughnut, right?

The pitcher plant—a deadly, meat-eating plant—is like a doughnut shop for insects.

You're an unsuspecting bug flying through the woods, and suddenly—yum!—something smells great.

You want a taste.

The smell is from a flower. *Perfect*—nectar is your favorite food!

To take a sip, you must fly inside the plant.

That's okay because you don't sense any danger.

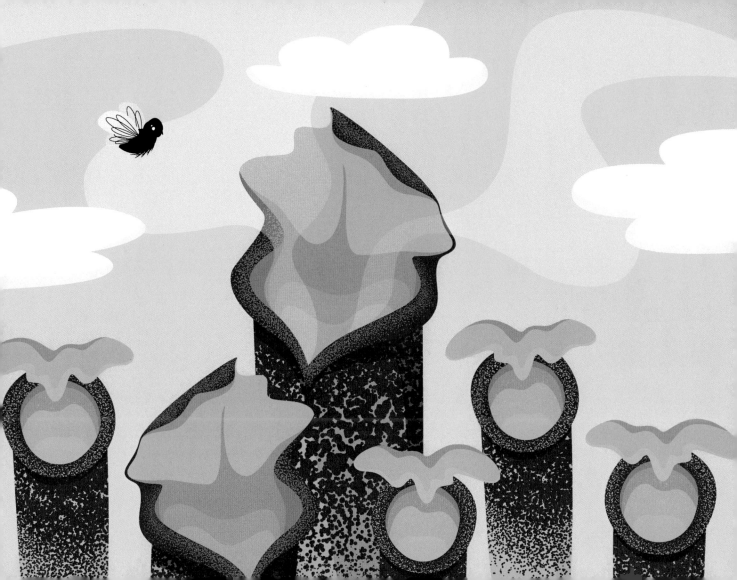

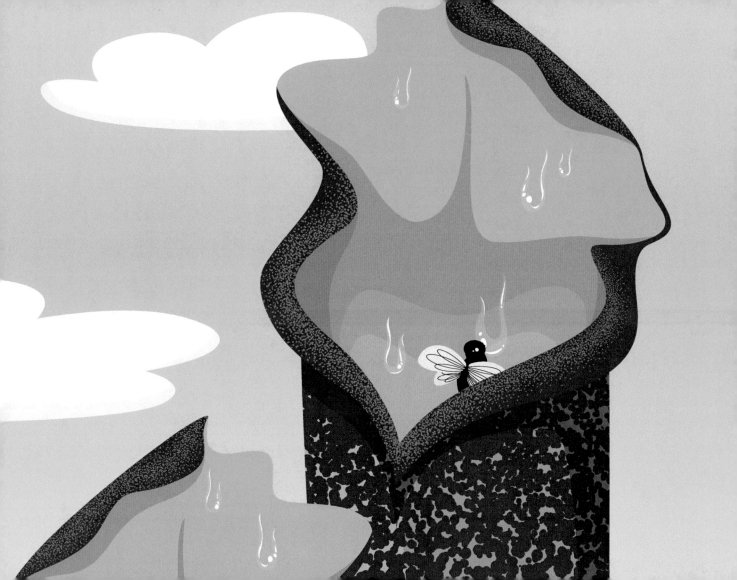

Yum! It's as good as it smells.

You don't notice how the plant is sloping under your feet, causing you to slide down a bit.

You're caught up in the moment—enjoying the sweet nectar treat.

You slide down a bit more.

That's kinda scary.

But you rationalize one more drink. After all, you have wings—you're fine.

You can fly out anytime.

You keep drinking because—even though you've had plenty—you also feel like you *need it*.

You aren't even really sure it tastes good anymore, but you *need just a few more sips*.

(Remember dopamine? Wanting but not liking?)

You're sliding down into the plant faster now.

The rim is farther and farther away.

You're a little freaked out, but another part of your brain says, "Don't worry, just a few more sips. You'll be fine."

You have wings, remember?

You can leave *anytime*.

You don't notice that your feet are now stuck.

You just need a few more sips.

You can handle it.

You can control it.

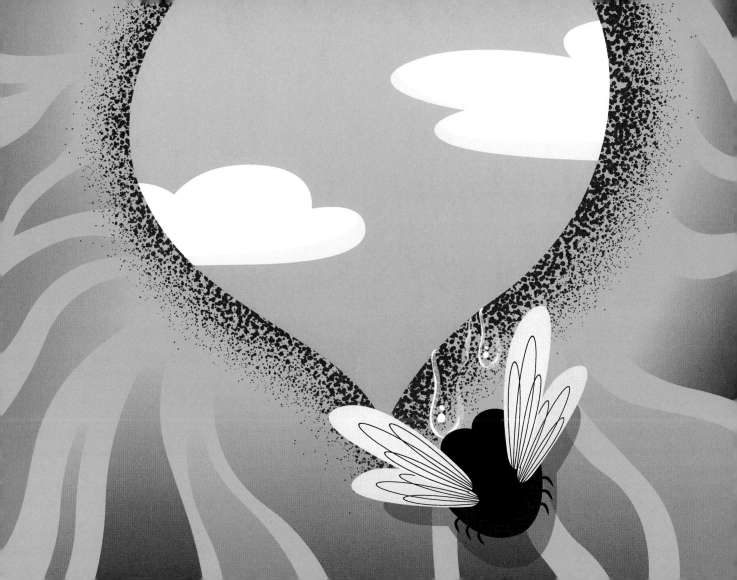

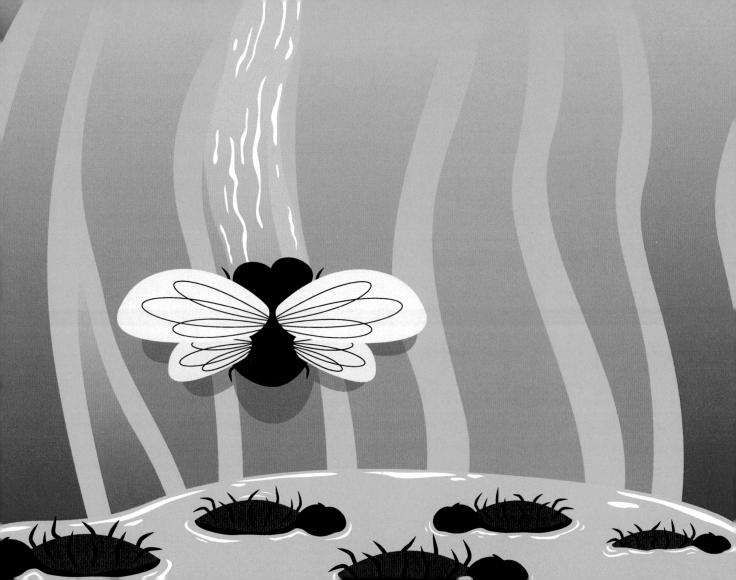

You can still leave at any time—at least, you hope so.

Suddenly, you are afraid.

You are at the bottom of the pitcher plant.

You stop drinking just long enough to notice the floating bodies of other bugs.

Bugs just like you.

You realize the nectar you can't get enough of is actually made from the bodies of other bugs, now dissolving in the juice.

Making the nectar.

You aren't *enjoying* the drink.

You are *becoming* the drink.

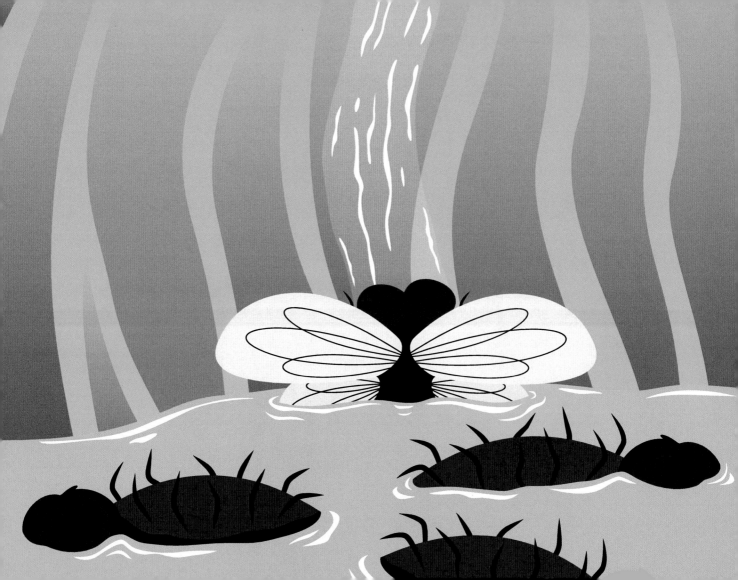

This is what the slide into alcohol is like.

It's slow.

It feels good at first.

You start to see warning signs but you think, "Not me. I'm in control. I have *wings*, after all."

But when it comes to alcohol, because of how the brain works, control is really hard.

You might wonder, "Can't we have the best of both worlds?"

Can't we enjoy the "nectar" just a little bit? And then fly away?

Maybe.

But maybe not.

Most people drink more—not less—over time.

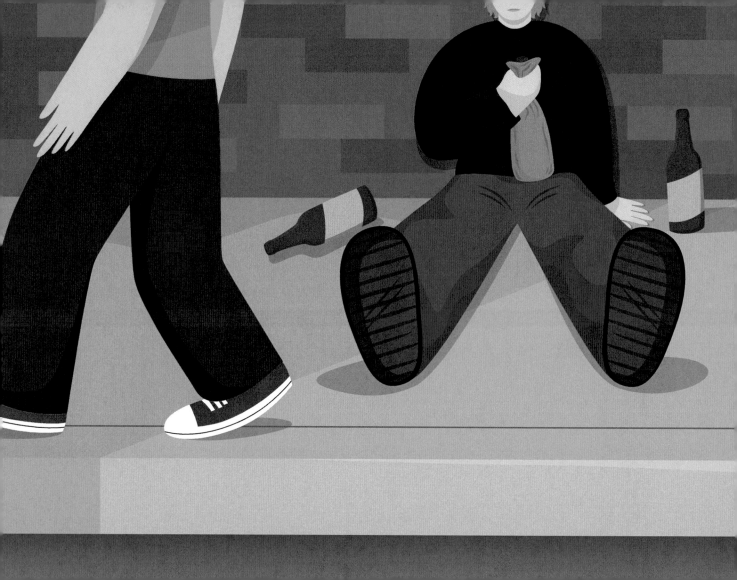

Basketball player Chris Herren—*who you should check out*—challenges us to think about this in another way.[10]

When you think about someone who's addicted to alcohol, someone stuck in the pitcher plant, what do you imagine?

Someone who's out of control? Who's lost everything? Someone pitiful?

We imagine the end stages when we think about an alcohol (or drug) problem.

The bottom of the pitcher plant.

But what about the first day?

The first drink?

The first sip?

What did someone—who is now in trouble with alcohol—look like when they were a kid?

Or a teenager?

They probably didn't look all that different from your friends.

Or you.

Or me.

And that's something I wish I had known before I had my first drink.

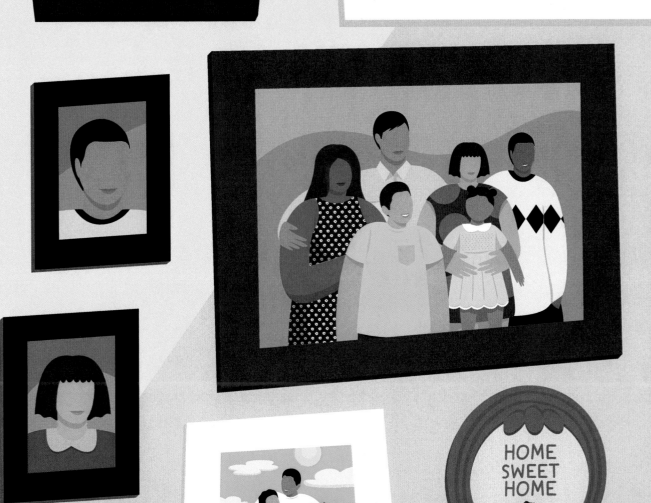

APPENDIX:
BUT WAIT, SO MANY QUESTIONS!

Q: Why do my parents drink? In fact, why does anyone drink?

A: There are so many reasons people drink. Since most of Western society drinks, it is seen as normal to do so and not normal to say no to alcohol. Also, alcohol does certain things that feel good in the moment; for instance, it slows your brain synapses so you actually think slower. Alcohol numbs the senses, dulling both physical and emotional pain. In fact, it was used in surgery in the 19th century, until we found safer options.[11]

This can feel like relief when your brain is overactive. Unfortunately, it also releases stress hormones so the result is more anxiety (feeling worried and/or agitated), not more relaxation. In addition, it gives you a euphoric (happy) feeling, like we talked about in the chapter "An Unfair Trade," but when the feeling wears off, it leaves you feeling worse than before.

Drinking generally starts because almost everyone around us is doing it. When we first drink, we probably don't like the taste, or even the feelings of dizziness or numbness, but alcohol is an addictive substance. The brain gets confused and we want to have more of it.

And before we know it, we may be drinking more than we intended. This can become a very slippery (dangerous) slope. The problem is that there is not a lot of information about some of the downsides of alcohol, so lots of people who are drinking more than they want to don't even realize that it is not entirely done by choice.

Q: I thought only "alcoholics" can get addicted to alcohol?

A: This is common knowledge (meaning most people believe it but don't question whether it's true), and like many things that are common knowledge, it needs to be looked at more closely. The truth is that the term *alcoholic* is no longer medically or scientifically agreed upon. There is no group of humans who become addicted to alcohol simply because of their genetics or their *"addictive personality."* All doctors, scientists, and medical professionals agree that *alcohol is addictive*. Not just to some people, but with the right amounts and frequency under the right circumstances—to all people. This, of course, has us wondering why isn't everyone addicted? In fact, many people are on the slippery slope toward addiction and don't realize it. There are many other reasons, and if you want to explore this great question further, please check out my book *This Naked Mind*.

Q: What is alcohol, exactly?

A: Alcohol has a few different forms but the one we drink is called ethanol. Interestingly, in many parts of the world, gasoline is also made of ethanol. The chemical compound for ethanol—both the kind in a car's gas tank and in a drinking glass—is C_2H_5OH. The actual chemical compound found in alcoholic drinks is very toxic (dangerous), and that is why we throw up if we drink too much. It is literally your body saving your life from the toxicity of the alcohol. And drinking just a small amount of pure alcohol would kill you, not to mention taste horrible. In fact, we have to use extensive distilling processes or mix alcohol with sugary liquids in order to make it taste good enough to drink. Another fascinating fact is that if animals are offered alcohol, they *will not* drink it—their instincts tell them it is poisonous. But we override our instincts by telling ourselves we just need to acquire the taste and that, because almost everyone else is doing it, alcohol must not be that bad.

Q: Can I try it and still be safe?

A: The best way to be safe when trying an alcoholic drink for the first time is to be well educated about alcohol. Most of us know more about the side effects of over-the-counter medicine like cough syrup than we do about alcohol. If we were all more informed about the harm that alcohol can cause, its addictive nature, and the signs of drinking too much, we could really improve our collective relationship with alcohol.

Q: What about peer pressure? Life is hard enough. If I choose not to drink, how will I fit in?

A: I spent a lot of time trying to fit in. I think we all do. And it wasn't until I decided to be true to myself that I really became "popular." People respect people who take a stand (as long as they do it without making anyone else feel bad). I know it's hard to believe, but by saying no, you actually do everyone around you a favor—you give them permission to say no as well. Which is probably what they want to do anyway. To practically navigate the situations, here are a few tips.

- Already have a drink in your hand—it doesn't matter that there isn't any alcohol in it, people don't really notice what you are drinking as long as you are drinking something.

- Since saying no can feel uncomfortable, say yes instead. When someone asks you if you want a drink, say "Yes, do you have any soda?"

- When others judge you or try and pressure you, realize that it's really about them, not you.

Q: What is so magic about the age 21 that makes it okay to drink? And why is the age different in other parts of the world?

A: There are different beliefs about when the brain will be less affected by alcohol. All experts agree that drinking while pregnant is harmful to the fetus and that drinking during childhood can negatively affect brain development.

Legal drinking ages began to take hold with some thought to when it would be "safer" to drink alcohol. Those ages have only increased over the years. In fact, between 1947 and 2014, many states in the US raised the drinking age from 18 to 21. Sadly, this was in response to how many people were being hurt or killed from drunk driving.

Although not many people know it, there is no truly safe amount of alcohol for any person, no matter their age.[12] That being said, the less developed the brain is, the harder it is to cope with alcohol, and most scientists agree that the human brain is not fully developed until the age of 25. Which, of course, has us wondering why 25 isn't the legal age. The truth is, the drinking age is somewhat random, and humans at any age should be very careful when drinking alcohol.

NEXT STEPS AND RECOMMENDED RESOURCES

If you want to learn more about alcohol and its relationship with the brain, I have multiple books that go deep into these topics. As of publication, these books have sold close to a million copies, been translated into multiple languages, and are available in many countries around the world.

For the most complete information, pick up a copy of *This Naked Mind* from any online bookstore (or visit ThisNakedMind.com for free resources).

If you or someone you know is interested in a 30-day Alcohol-Free Challenge, you can grab a copy of *The Alcohol Experiment* from an online bookstore. Or join us for our Free Alcohol Experiment at AlcoholExperiment.com.

And if you would rather listen to podcasts, check out *This Naked Mind* podcast wherever you get your podcasts. *This Naked Mind* is the top podcast on this topic, and as of publication, is ranked in the top 1% of all podcasts globally, with more than 500 episodes.

NOTES

1   *The Addictive Brain* by Thad A. Polk is the main resource for this book.

2   Terry E. Robinson and Kent C. Berridge, "The Incentive Sensitization Theory of Addiction: Some Current Issues," *Philosophical Transactions of the Royal Society B*, July 18, 2008, doi.org/10.1098/rstb.2008.0093.

3   Marisa Roberto and Nicholas W. Gilpin, "Central Amygdala Neuroplasticity in Alcohol Dependence," *Neurobiology of Alcohol Dependence*, 2014, sciencedirect.com/topics/neuroscience/dynorphin.

4   David H. Jernigan, "The Extent of Global Alcohol Marketing and Its Impact on Youth," *Contemporary Drug Problems*, 2010, doi.org/10.1177/009145091003700104.

5   Mandy Stahre, PhD, MPH; Jim Roeber, MSPH; Dafna Kanny, PhD; Robert D. Brewer, MD, MSPH; Xingyou Zhang, PhD, "Contribution of Excessive Alcohol Consumption to Deaths and Years of Potential Life Lost in the United States," *Preventing Chronic Disease*, June 26, 2014, dx.doi.org/10.5888/pcd11.130293.

6   "2013 Mortality Multiple Cause Micro-data Files," US Centers for Disease Control (Atlanta, GA), December 2014, Table 10, pp. 19–23, cdc.gov/nchs/nvss/mortality_public_use_data.htm.

7   "Blood Alcohol Levels and You," Eastern Kentucky University Counseling Center, counselingcenter.eku.edu/blood-alcohol-levels-and-you.

8   Christoph Schwarzer, "30 Years of Dynorphins – New Insights on Their Functions in Neuropsychiatric Diseases," *Pharmacology & Therapeutics*, 2009, ncbi.nlm.nih.gov/pmc/articles/PMC2872771.

9   Allison T. Knoll and William A. Carlezon, Jr., "Dynorphin, Stress, and Depression," *Brain Research*, 2010, ncbi.nlm.nih.gov/pmc/articles/PMC2819644.

10 herrentalks.com and thisnakedmind.com/ep-463-the-first-day-with-chris-herren.

11 Mallery True, "Alcoholism: From Past to Present," Indiana University School of Medicine, March 8, 2019, medicine.iu.edu/blogs/medical-library/historical-book-of-the-week-effects-of-alcoholic-drinks-tobacco-sedatives-1949.

12 Anya Topiwala, Klaus P. Ebmeier, Thomas Maullin-Sapey, and Thomas E. Nichols, "No Safe Level of Alcohol Consumption for Brain Health: Observational Cohort Study of 25,378 UK Biobank Participants," medRxiv, 2021, medrxiv.org/content/10.1101/2021.05.10.21256931v1.

ABOUT THE AUTHOR

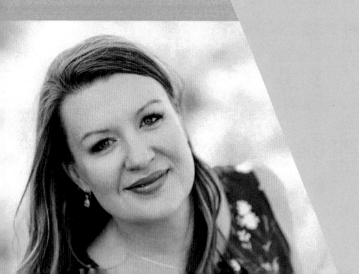

Annie Grace is the author of *This Naked Mind: Control Alcohol, Find Freedom, Discover Happiness & Change Your Life* and *The Alcohol Experiment: A 30-Day, Alcohol-Free Challenge to Interrupt Your Habits and Help You Take Control*. She grew up outside Aspen, Colorado, in a one-room log cabin without running water or electricity. Having discovered a passion for marketing, Annie Grace earned a master of science in marketing and dove into corporate life.

As the youngest vice president in a multinational company at the age of 26, her drinking career began in earnest. At 35, in a global C-level marketing role, she was responsible for marketing in 28 countries; she was drinking almost 2 bottles of wine a night. Knowing she needed a change but unwilling to submit to a life of deprivation and stigma, Annie Grace embarked on a journey to painlessly gain control of alcohol—for her that process resulted in no longer wanting to drink. Never happier, she left her executive role to write and share *This Naked Mind* with the world.

In her free time, she loves to ski, travel (26 countries and counting), and enjoy her beautiful family. Annie Grace lives with her husband and 3 children in the Colorado mountains.

Made in the USA
Monee, IL
12 November 2022

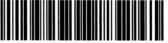

17568645R00069